Lifting The WEIGHT

THE JOURNEY TO TOTAL FREEDOM

PRESENTED BY SHERELL BROWN

Presented By Sherell Brown

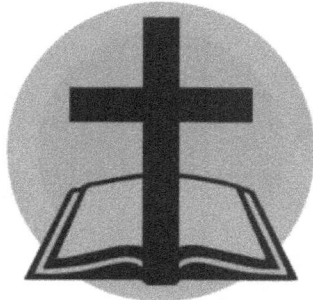

Lifting the Weight
The Journey to Total Freedom

Presented By
Sherell Brown

Pearly Gates
Publishing LLC
"Inspiring Christian Authors to BE Authors"
Pearly Gates Publishing LLC™, Houston, Texas

Lifting the Weight: The Journey to Total Freedom

Lifting the Weight
The Journey to Total Freedom

ISBN 10: 1945117761
ISBN 13: 9781945117763
Library of Congress Control Number: 2017942407

For information and bulk ordering, contact:
Pearly Gates Publishing LLC
Angela R. Edwards, CEO
P.O. Box 62287
Houston, TX 77205
BestSeller@PearlyGatesPublishing.com

Presented By Sherell Brown

DEDICATION

Lifting the Weight is dedicated to all of the people out there who are on the relentless pursuit of their destiny.

Life will try to throw **everything** at you - including the kitchen sink - but you have to *know* you have the ability to rise up and overcome. You will face rejection. You will question your relevance. Rest assured, however: **The world needs your resilience.** This is not the time to pull back; it's time to push forward. Take ownership of your gifts and place your stake in the ground as we work *together* to take back your territory.

Where are all of my overcomers, sickness-tried, obesity-tried, divorce-tried, abuse-tried, and family-tried? Guess what? **You're still standing!** It's not that you never fought a battle. It's not the fact that you carry scars. Rather, it is the fact that you *never stopped.*

You *never stopped* pushing. You *never stopped* fighting. You **never** gave up.

Even when they were "preaching the benediction" over your life, **GOD** was speaking resurrection power into you. Your life is a testament…each day a page…each year a chapter. That is why the weight must be lifted. That is why you must walk in **TOTAL** freedom. The world awaits your greatness!

The pages of your life must be read
so that other souls can be fed.

ACKNOWLEDGMENTS

First, giving honor and glory to God from whom **all** blessings flow.

I would like to thank my family for their continued support in the execution of the vision to take the message of healing, health, and hope around the world.

To my husband, Desmond Brown: I thank you for your never-ending support.

To my beautiful children: Mommy loves you.

To each of the Co-Authors: You are beautiful, brave women who answered the call and have bared their souls in the pages to come. I am forever grateful and the world is forever blessed because you did not hold to the hurt of the past. You are now empowered and propelled by your past, doing just what the Word declares: setting the captives free.

To our Publisher, Mrs. Angela Edwards: Thank you for your continued support throughout the journey and for being a part of bringing this baby to life.

To each and every one of you who have supported the vision of *Lifting the Weight*: We are forever grateful.

INTRODUCTION

This anthology is a celebration of triumph over tragedy. You are encouraged to trust your process. What a privilege it is to bring you experts who poured from their lives and deposited sustaining stories for your journey forward. With transparency and integrity, they share the weights they carried for years and the systems they used to lift them - physical, mental, and emotional weights they were able to permanently remove from their lives.

The stories penned herein are not just raw and relatable; they equip you with tools you can reference time and again for your journey to acquire maximum results!

Lifting the Weight: The Journey to Total Freedom

TABLE OF CONTENTS

Presented By Sherell Brown

Don't Throw Away Your Notes
By Eboni Gee

In the beginning

"Lifting the weight" was my goal growing up at home. I grew up in a household with my mother, father, sister, and - *17 years later* - brother. My parents had trust, forgiveness, and relationship issues which trickled down to my siblings and me. I vividly remember my father bringing up old stories about what my mother did to him years ago (my mother had been deceptive about having my sister and brother, so the trust was no longer there). My father consistently lived in the past, so forgiveness was not there, either. Phony facades, angry whispers in public, and misery were all that was left in our home.

In my father's absence, we would listen to music, dance around, and have fun...all the while, staring out the window awaiting his inevitable return. Once my father pulled up, the fun was over and the gloom began. This started when I was six years old and lasted long after I moved out of the home at the age of 18.

My upbringing created bad coping skills, trust issues, and the inability to forgive. My mental health was deeply-scarred and grew progressively worse as I developed bad habits of my own. I couldn't develop and maintain relationships because I trusted **no one**. Those closest to me who wronged me were "*one and done*". Periodically, there were second chances given - with **no** room for error **nor** apology. The weight that accumulated because of my mindset was exhausting.

In my early 20s, I knew how I perceived my life and the people around me were flawed, so I started researching. I bought self-help books, prayed *really* hard, and genuinely wanted to change. Nothing happened. I couldn't understand it! I was doing "the work" (or so I thought)! ***Why wasn't change coming about?***

I didn't understand that I had to interpret the information I was reading. I had to create the goals and strategies of how I would implement and execute them. Finally, I needed to know what my outcomes were going to be.

How did I want to feel?

What did I want to accomplish?

How would these changes impact my life moving forward?

Those are the things books don't tell you. They give a *generalized* overview of what you need to do, but there is no personalized direction nor feedback for your **individual** path. Although I was aware I had mindset issues, I wasn't able to begin the work I needed to do to pull myself out of the hole I was living in…yet. I needed to dig deeper, but I didn't.

My Crossroad

I have always been externally self-motivated. I began to work on my issues on a superficial level. I focused my efforts on my physical wellness. What I didn't realize was that I was overcompensating for an area I could control for one I could not. Since I couldn't figure out how to heal mentally, I moved on to something that was "easy": I was an emotional-eater and had an unhealthy relationship with food.

I eventually found my sweet spot with weight loss and began to work out a couple of hours a day, three to five days a week. I was finally beginning to feel like I was living! Things were going great. I was engaged, super-fit, and back in school.

In 2004, my mother was diagnosed with Cancer. At the time, I was juggling working full time, going to school full time, saving to purchase a house, planning a wedding, and helping my mother. Helping my mother out during this time brought me back into a toxic space with my father. What little progress I made with my mindset felt like it was fading away. I realized I had never forgiven him for his actions when I was growing up. The anger I carried had always poisoned other areas of my life, but I never related the two. I surely couldn't deal with those thoughts and feelings at **THAT** moment, so I pushed them down and kept moving.

My mother fought a good fight, but she passed away two years after her diagnosis. After her passing, I never went back to resolve any of those old feelings, so they continued to fester...slowly infecting my mind.

As time went on, I had a son, took custody of my younger brother, and finished nursing school. Well, the weight came back...and then some. I still did not have the time to work on me - *at least that's what I told myself.*

Lifting the Weight: The Journey to Total Freedom

Many of the experiences I faced during this time added to and exacerbated my mental health. Dealing with the mental instabilities of others was hard on me. Life has a way of creating crossroads. I had arrived at my own. I started having bouts of light-headedness, nausea, shortness of breath, and increased heart rate. At first, I thought something was physically wrong with me. After seeing my doctor, it was determined I was suffering from anxiety. I had two options: take medication or change my lifestyle.

I opted to change my lifestyle.

I couldn't imagine taking pills to control something in my mind I could control on my own. I had to get **serious** about healing my mind and living the life I deserved.

The Phoenix Rises

My astrological sign is Gemini. Gemini is represented by twins. I call my "twin" 'Phoenix'. I kept her inside because she represented the side of me I fought to keep hidden. She personified the anger and rage I carried. She showed up strongly in one of my main issues: my inner-critic.

We all have an inner-critic that lives within. The inner-critic loves to blame, shame, and criticize you for decisions you made in the past and for all that has gone wrong in your life. Your inner-critic also causes you to judge yourself and others. Comparison - which steals your joy - is also a characteristic. Comparison destroys your self-confidence, self-esteem, and self-worth.

I had few meaningful relationships, which (in general) is not a problem. However, when you don't have the ability to foster meaningful relationships because of continually pushing people away and cutting them off, it's an unhealthy place to be.

My inner-critic also affected my internal motivation. Internally, I couldn't genuinely motivate myself because I had no idea what my *"WHY?"* was. I had to ask myself what I really wanted to do with my life and why I wanted to do it. In my case, my inner-critic manifested as unrealistic expectations about almost everything I couldn't control. It sabotaged most of my internal efforts! My inner-critic had a huge hold on me for many reasons.

Lifting the Weight: The Journey to Total Freedom

I didn't go straight to college right out of high school.

I made some poor decisions in the past and felt like I should have been further along in life.

I had to find what I called my "voice of positivity".

The voice of positivity is full of self-compassion, self-love, self-respect, and self-trust. I had to first be kind to myself, admit my shortcomings, and then resolve them. I had to forgive myself for everything, no matter what the circumstances were. I had to adapt to a mindset that was positive, grateful, and healthy. I had to heal my mind and nurture my emotional, mental, and spiritual growth. Forgiveness of others was needed, too; but until I forgave myself, I didn't know what that looked like. I had to love me, no matter what the scale read. I had to care for me, even when I fell short of my expectations. The person I became because of the transformation was worth all of the sacrifices, tears, and frustrations.

YES:
There will be sacrifices throughout the process.

I had to dig in and connect to myself in a way I never had before. It required me being still and quieting my mind so that I could gain clarity on what it was that haunted me. I needed to receive answers. Before, my prayers consisted of asking for a way out of the mess, but my mind was so cluttered, I was unable to hear the response.

The process was not something I did a few times and then forgot about. It is a **lifestyle change** - one I built on a strong foundation and allowed it to evolve my mindset with past successes, challenges, and lessons. I learned how to cope with life in a healthy way. It feels good and natural to me. I became a master at guarding and filtering what I allowed to enter my mind. I became more aware of my triggers and planned how I would counter them. I acquired the skill of testing my perception of life against the facts. There was no more making assumptions and living in a reality that was skewed by my emotions.

Lifting the Weight: The Journey to Total Freedom

I had to learn that my thoughts created feelings, and those feelings created behaviors. If I was in a negative thought pattern, everything that resulted was negative - which produced undesired effects in my life. By adopting a positive "self", my patterns became positive and my life changed. I still needed to keep digging to unlock the key to my healing and learn how to apply what I learned to my life...*permanently*.

My Healing

The first thing I did was conduct a deep self-reflection. We heal in layers, so the first layer I peeled back was "addressing me". I went way back and reconciled all of the trouble spots. This process was very time-consuming. I had to confront all of the ugly truths I had been running from: unresolved issues, people I needed to forgive, managing my expectations, learning how to have a better relationship with food, and losing weight. I also realized I lost my joy after six straight years in school, being a wife and mother, and working full time. I didn't have **any** activities I did just for me.

Worse yet, I had no idea what I enjoyed doing anymore!

After my reflection, I wrote a list of all of the things I needed to do and crossed them off as I completed them. As I stated earlier, this, too, took time to accomplish. I processed through each thought and feeling I had, understanding why I had them, and then closed the chapter. I had a bad habit of reliving my past and its associated pain.

To truly move on and be present in life, reliving the past is not an option. You must let it go.

Once the chains that were holding me back were broken, I came up with a game plan to support my positive mindset, heal, and focus on wellness in other areas of my life. This is where self-care and personal development came into play.

Lifting the Weight: The Journey to Total Freedom

I started researching things I enjoyed doing. This was very important. Having an outlet where I could unplug and have some fun was essential to my healing. I also started meditating, journaling, and having devotional time daily. This kept my mind from racing, my thoughts positive, and my mindset focused on growth. I became more intentional with reading books that would help me in some way. When I read developmental books in the past, I didn't have the foundation needed to apply what they were "speaking" into my life. Personal development is trial and error. Every suggestion will not work for everyone. I had to try many different solutions and find what worked best for me. I had to figure out how to consistently live the life I wanted, all while living in a world of unknown outcomes. The art of 'allowing' came into my life, and it was just what I needed to accomplish the goal.

'Allowing' is when you accept the things that happen in your life - both the good and the bad. Instead of fighting for control, you become open to life and embrace the lessons that arrive. The premise of 'allowing' is to free yourself and let what is supposed to happen occur.

Life is about harmony and growth. If we don't stretch, we will never grow. Instead, the restriction leaves us stuck and complaining about the same things over and over again. We will continue to stay in the box we have built for ourselves and never expand our ability to handle different experiences. Trust is required. You must believe all things are working for your good.

This way of thinking opened me up to a whole new world of multiple possibilities - and **JOY**! I *allowed* myself to be present in my journey and take things as they came. I no longer stressed about what happened in the past. I no longer stressed about those things to come, either. I stayed mindful and participated in my experiences, which brought so much joy to my life. I let go of controlling ways in my life that didn't serve me. I had regained my freedom. It was then I lost the mental, emotional, and psychological weights.

Lifting the Weight: The Journey to Total Freedom

My Strategy

After my healing came preparation. I had developed anxiety because I always needed to be in control while worrying about the outcome if I was not. When faced with a life-altering decision of learning how to forgive or lose a dear relationship, I sprang into action. I chose to treat my anxiety with diet and exercise. I developed a plan that would nurture my growth and continue to strengthen my mind. Doing so began the healing of my body. Self-awareness is key at this stage. Being aware of your triggers, how you respond to situations, and how you want to show up will guide you as you work on improving your life and living a healthy lifestyle.

I picked out my favorite Bible verses and affirmations, made a folder in the notes section of my phone, and wrote them all down. When you get into the thick of things, you don't want to find yourself having to think about what your next move is going to be. *Preparation* was key to my success. When I began to feel anxious, I recited something I had written down. I picked whatever best suited me in the moment.

In the beginning, I was very sensitive, so I was triggered easily and often. As time passed (and with practice), I was able to grow stronger and use this technique less. I read the book *The Miracle Morning* by Hal Elrod (if you have never read it, I suggest you do). That book added structure to my strategy. I was already doing most of the **S.A.V.E.R.S.** (Silence; Affirmations; Visualization; Exercise; Reading; Scribing). The book gave me organization and a routine to follow.

For one hour in the morning, I spend time in silence, saying affirmations, visualizing what I desire, exercising, reading, and journaling. With this routine, I created healthy habits that increased my self-discipline, willpower, and consistency. I had time to discover who I was and practiced being mindful daily. Through my devotionals, faith, and trust in myself, my path was restored. I had to believe what I wanted was 100% possible for me to do and achieve. I spend time every day seeing myself achieving my goals and living in my purpose. I develop the feelings my success will bring and pray for clarity to direct me.

Lifting the Weight: The Journey to Total Freedom

My Action

Taking action activates your strategy. Your plan will do you **no** good if you never act on it. Many things can cause inaction: fear, self-doubt, and procrastination - just to name a few. I *could have* let life keep me inactivated. I *could have* used the excuse of it being too hard and complicated. On the contrary, I **embraced** the complicated. It has taught me so many lessons about resilience and bravery. Life being complicated isn't what throws us off-track; it's our response to the complication.

Oftentimes, we choose to operate in a problem-focused mindset. When we do that, our focus is on what's wrong instead of finding a solution. When we shift to a solution-focused mindset, we put all of our efforts into solving our problems in a positive, constructive way. The positivity you have brings energy that creates favor in your life.

Let go of perfection. Nothing will ever be perfect. All you can do is turn your lessons into blessings and keep moving forward. Live courageously, which is action despite fear. You will never feel absolutely ready to begin this journey. Waiting for readiness is just another way for fear to control you and keep you from taking action. Action is the phase where the weight-loss begins. By putting my strategy into action, I was finally able to heal my mind, release the weight, and live in my purpose of helping others press through the fear and pursue their hearts' desires.

Conclusion

In conclusion, I will say this: **Stop waiting on permission to go after your dreams.** Start praying and asking for what you want. Believe that what you want will undoubtedly happen for you. Start living every single day with gratitude and watch your desires come to life.

I used to be a skeptic of manifestation and visualization, but once I experienced the process, I was hooked!

Lifting the Weight: The Journey to Total Freedom

Once you have accomplished defining your goals, defining your blocks, and putting a plan in place to resolve them, you are ready to manifest your vision. Take the vision for your life that you have created and begin to focus your energies and thoughts towards that life. Every morning, spend at least five minutes actively thinking about how your life will be when your vision happens.

Thoughts become things. When you shift your thinking to be productive, **AMAZING** things will start happening in your life.

Now, you are human. Those negative thoughts will creep in from time to time. A great way to check in with your thoughts is to pay close attention to how you are feeling. Often, your feelings will be more noticeable than the fact that your thoughts have went south. Keep the positivity flowing to keep your thoughts in check. Create ways to keep yourself present and focused on your result. You will only go as high as your thoughts can take you, so I ask: *How high are your dreams? How will you expand your life this year?* Pursuing your goals and dreams requires massive personal development because it's parallel to your success. Growth and continual learning are parts of life. You can never learn too much.

You will still have "bad" days. You will find yourself wanting to give up. You will get frustrated. The difference is now you have the tools, techniques, and skills to bounce back quickly. Ultimately, how you respond will be up to you. The truth is this: Until we are faced with these difficult times in life, we never know how we will respond. Stop living in the shadows of fear and self-doubt. Commit to start writing a new chapter in your life - one filled with self-compassion, forgiveness, and joy. The grass grows where you water it. Take the time to nurture your mental, emotional, and spiritual health so that your physical health can follow. Lose your inner-critic and find power and strength in your voice of positivity.

I realized that in order to get my life to a place of unconditional peace and happiness, I had to heal my mind *AND* body. I also had to nourish my spirit and strengthen my mind. All of these pieces worked together in awesome harmony to create the person I am today.

Lifting the Weight: The Journey to Total Freedom

This lifestyle isn't something you do one time and set aside; you must *continuously* work at maintaining a positive outlook on life, have positive coping skills, and be content where you are. For me, I know that has always been a challenge. I love to be in control and even though I know I am not, that doesn't stop the need to have control. Every day, I work on myself - not only to shake the "control bug", but also to understand why I have that need.

To overcome obstacles in your way and move on to making goals that set you on the true course of your purpose, you must deal with why you have those obstacles. If you don't, they will show up in the most unlikely places. When that happens, it will eat away at your confidence, create self-doubt, and smother your dreams. Many people never recover from this because they just don't know how to deal with their issues in healthy ways.

The words you speak to yourself.
The foods you consume.
The peace that can only come from within.

Those three areas work together to create a harmonious way of life and make this *phenomenal* experience one you get to live every day. They provide a choice of how to live and sets you on a course to take care of your own well-being.

Truly Healing the Weight
By Iris Hernandez

It all started with perfection and the idea that the body is supposed to be a certain way. As you go through an eating disorder, emotional stability is definitely not what you think about or connect to your imbalance. **Trust me: I know.** The constant battle with Anorexia and Bulimia had me completely blind. I had the connection to basic emotions such as happiness, anger, jealousy, and disappointment; however, I did not know there were deeper emotions I needed to watch out for - or that the emotions would actually become trapped in my body and subconscious mind.

As you may already know, I am an advocate for health and healing. However, during a few years of my life, I became stuck in my body. Self-image was all that occupied my mind. Have you ever felt that way? It was like a strong bondage and no matter what I did, my relationship with food was the worst. I saw food as an enemy. I thought food was the reason the problems in my body kept reoccurring. I believed I could not have the perfect image because of my food choices.

As I began to break free, food was no longer my worst enemy. My own thoughts and emotions took the "worst enemy" spot. I began to realize the truth about healing, the power that emotions hold, and the reason why people have such a hard time breaking free from illness. It was no longer just about an eating disorder; it became about broken hearts (Isaiah 61:1).

In this chapter, I will discuss three major parts to healing and **truly** lifting the weight. We will begin with blindness, follow with recognition, and lastly, touch bases on a few things that can help you with the healing journey. I will also share a few scriptures which have helped change my life. I pray this chapter changes someone's view about her body, overall way of thinking, and definitely the way we treat and see our brothers and sisters, as we never know the hidden pain within.

Blindness

There may be a point in your life when you block thoughts, events, and emotions. This often happens during childhood, but it is not limited to that period in life. I have worked with adults who put themselves to sleep after a major event or crisis - usually a loved-one's death or experience with major abuse. I have also noticed recurring emotions will build up and cause great imbalances.

You may be asking, *"Put themselves to sleep?"* Yes. That is exactly what I call it: Sleep-walkers (to be specific) because those people are unconsciously still functioning in their daily routines. They go to work, spend time with family, etc., but they have decided to 'check out' emotionally. If the emotional pain is bad enough, they may even begin to stop recognizing changes in their body. The changes may not be noticed unless there is a great deal of pain attached to the change, which is (in my opinion) a very dangerous thing. Pain or discomfort (as you may already know) is a mechanism that allows us to recognize a weakness or problem in our body. A lack of awareness closes our intuition. When there is a loss of connection, blindness begins.

Blindness is just that: an inability to see. For this part of my journey, it was the inability to **feel**. There is such a thing as emotional blindness. We call it unconsciousness, which can actually lead to reproductive system imbalances such as endometriosis, prostate trouble, ovarian cysts, tumors, irregular cycles, low testosterone, and more. Trapped emotions can truly wreak major havoc in the body, even to the point of affecting the hair and skin. The sad thing is that we are at a point in society where we feel the need to simply remove the blinders instead of opening our eyes to deeper levels of healing. It's another level of social blindness or unawareness. I could even say a numbness to the hurt that is disrupting the world. We are all one (Romans 12:5); every decision made can be felt by all. That is why awareness or opening of the eyes is so important (Acts 26:18). In that way, we can step fully into light and see farther than what is in front of us - even to the point of seeing your full potential or finally getting to the point of reaching your goals and fulfilling your dreams. That is what **true** healing is about.

Lifting the Weight: The Journey to Total Freedom

So, what does this have to do with the weight-loss journey? **EVERYTHING!** True healing should not only be physical. The blindness can lead to a broken heart. Think about it: When we do not love ourselves enough to stop abusing our own bodies, there is a great chance that a broken heart may be involved. A broken heart is not just about sadness; a broken heart is a broken soul…a broken spirit - something which the media is becoming aware of.

Every organ in your body has emotional connections or reactions. I will discuss them later in the chapter, but the *heart* is where the majority of them are stored (Proverbs 4:23). So, keep in mind: blindness is **not** just about the eyes. Allow your *spiritual* eyes to be opened and, in turn, begin to recognize the deeper connection between soul and body (Genesis 2:7).

Recognition

We are composed of three parts: spirit, soul, and body (1 Thessalonians 5:23), with the soul being composed of thoughts and emotions. Thoughts and emotions are the most deceitful because they can guide your every step. Most of the healing must happen on a soul level. Remember: *There is a difference between healing and simply having a healthy body.* Both of them are important, but when we care only for our body, it can be a temporary fix. We must, in turn, care for our soul so that the spirit can shine through.

Have you ever seen a super-happy person? A person who just *RADIATES*? That is what a clean spirit looks like. I have noticed healthy-looking people who do not have **THAT** glow. So, the goal is the realization - the awareness - of what we are composed of. The goal is to reach happiness and self-love (Mark 12:31).

Back to the soul...

Lifting the Weight: The Journey to Total Freedom

Remember I mentioned the soul can guide our every step? That's because the heart is involved. Did you grow up hearing, "Follow your heart"? I did. No one ever told me that if I was not in *Christ*, my heart would be the most deceitful of all things (Jeremiah 17:9). No one ever told me that if I followed my heart, I could actually end up in big trouble...and I did. I'm not talking about just a broken relationship, but also with many bad decisions which impacted my life and body. Healing from those negative decisions still affects me after many years. It was a heaviness added to my soul. I remember storing tons of guilt and lack of forgiveness towards myself. In turn, I either over-ate or under-ate.

The worst part about it was the lack of awareness. I did not know I was lacking self-forgiveness; therefore, I remained in physical, psychological, and emotional pain. It was such a strange place to be, especially because there seemed to be certain pieces missing. It all just feels like heaviness...like depression...like there is no way out. It's like that certain place in life where nothing nor anything can move you. It's the feeling of being overwhelmed and alone. It has to be the deepest and worst point - the turning point - when you realize that is where the healing begins.

Presented By Sherell Brown

Recognize where you are and, at times, ask for help.

I thank **GOD** for positive people, positive thoughts, and encouragement. Realize positivism is amazingly powerful. That is why positive thoughts, emotions, relationships, and decisions can bring your healing journey into an incredible speed (Proverbs 23:7). So, the healing journey took me into a deeper awareness on how to recognize and eventually replace emotions. I found a few techniques (to be discussed in the next section) that worked great, but I realized healing power is much greater than those things that are tangible.

So, to sum this section up: Remember, being aware of the information should allow for you to view yourself as more than just a physical body. In that way, we can stop focusing only on the physical body and move on to cleansing our **WHOLE** selves. Remember, being completely focused on the body can happen in such a subtle way that you may be able to notice the imbalance once out and set free. That is why we need to make sure recognition is something everyone becomes aware of at all times. Take the information as gifts and opportunities to become better.

Lifting the Weight: The Journey to Total Freedom

It starts with focus and questioning of feelings and thoughts. In creating a union with self, the development of a relationship with self is the same as that with a friend or loved-one. Developing a true union with self can be a bit difficult at first, but it all begins with acceptance which, believe it or not, is a great emotion for healing eating disorders.

Tools for the Healing Journey

The best and initial way of working with trapped emotions or lifting the weight is by self-expression. This may be difficult at first, especially since most people actually do a fantastic job at swallowing true feelings or emotions - such as when we have a lot we would love to express (especially to the person who may need to hear it), but at the perfect time, only silence comes out. At this point, writing is best...honest writing. I say 'honest' because there are times when ever our "personal" journals do not receive our full truths. If possible, write daily. This part is so important for your freedom because it teaches you how to get closer to who you are. It gives the outlet - the way for you to create and remove whatever you want.

Once you are ready, you can move on to freestyle painting, singing, and even dancing! The last two allow for the body to release trapped emotions. Trapped emotions can truly harm the body. Weight loss is not limited; it is simply years of packed away emotions, thoughts, ideas, and/or tears. I know for a fact this is true because I have seen people lose 25-30 pounds in a crazy-fast speed simply by releasing secrets or trapped words.

This part of the chapter is titled "Tools"; therefore, I must give you the tools I used to achieve this type of release. Like anything else, it requires some practice. *Please keep that in mind.*

I wanted to take a moment to mention the "Emotional Code Chart". I would love to give credit to the creator of such an amazing chart: Dr. Bradley Nelson. Every cell in our body has a memory. Even our skin will forever remember touches or mistreatment. Experts say this is all stored in our subconscious mind. Clearing is all about moving forward, so the big point here is walking in faith (2 Corinthians 5:7). There is a difference between having the tools and actually using them (James 2:17).

Lifting the Weight: The Journey to Total Freedom

You have received the initial steps toward breaking free - the steps toward a different kind of health and healing. Remember: We are more than just a physical body. When we remember such, then we can take the steps toward making changes. The most important of all the tools is the realization that we are on a spiritual journey. I know and understand not everyone can receive scripture the same way or that there may be different points of view; however, based off of life's experiences in all levels of health and healing, I can honestly say scripture and my choice to focus on Christ has completely rerouted my life for the better. I say all of that because I want to mention how important prayer is for healing. Prayer changes things, and I noticed how praying before eating made the biggest change of all. It allowed me to become one with my food and not see it as an enemy. I now see food for what it is purposed: *nourishment*.

I often tell my clients, "*While praying, say, **"I am worthy to receive goodness and life"**"*. In that way, you consciously recognize your food choices while at the same time, know that prayer has changed **everything** - as well as your overall ability to receive and know you are worthy.

It is all about the walk with faith. Don't forget to pray for the desire to love healthy and nutritious foods for your body because we are all so different and in different places in our journey of life. Health is not cookie cutter-style, so rearrange accordingly and, most importantly, be patient and loving to yourself.

Conclusion

In conclusion, healing is a journey. This particular journey is not only about self-healing, but also about the healing of our global community. When we are individually out of balance, we are the representation of the illness seen in the world. However, when we choose to better our situation, we also choose to better the world. We begin to care not only for ourselves, but also about our community - about our brothers and sisters (1 John 3:16). When you heal, we all heal. It's as simple as that.

This is such an amazing journey, but only you can take the first step. Remember: In order for the journey to begin, we must first remove the blindfold, recognize the steps of healing, and finally, use the tools to turn a broken heart into a whole and complete heart (Ezekiel 36:26).

Lifting the Weight: The Journey to Total Freedom

I know this book is more about weight loss, but being a Holistic Practitioner and with emotions being my favorite part of healing, I cannot limit my chapter or categorize. The healing journey is abundant, constant, and never-ending. A certain beauty is contained therein that helps you reach more levels of self-awareness and love. I pray this chapter changes your perspective towards yourself and that you will treat your spirit, soul, and body with compassion and respect - past, present, and future.

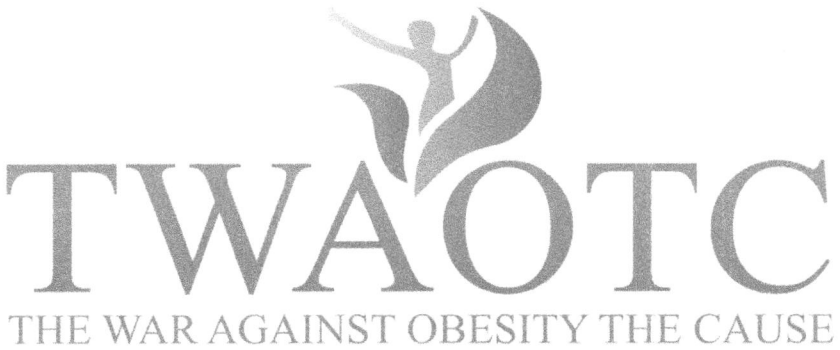

TWAOTC
THE WAR AGAINST OBESITY THE CAUSE

The Journey to Total Freedom
By Sherell Brown

"Come unto me, all ye that labor and are heavy laden, and I will give
you rest. Take my yoke upon you, and learn of me;
for I am meek and lowly in heart:
and ye shall find rest unto your souls"
(Matthew 11:28-30).

There was an exchange on Calvary paid for with the blood of Jesus, and because His precious blood was shed, it is our **birthright** to live and be free - free in mind, body, and soul. However, as we know, life is filled with circumstances and situations that will shake our very core beliefs. It's up to us to not allow it to happen.

See, what I understood is that when this exchange happened, I was given divine health, abundance, joy, love, peace, and all I could ever think or imagine. If you were to assess your life right now and find that you are coming up short, that means *something* is trying to take what rightfully belongs to you. Here is one thing I want you to remember: **We are not fighting to gain something. We are fighting to keep what is ours.**

When you do not understand who you are and the authority you possess, only then what is yours can be stolen. Today, I come to tell you that freedom can be yours in every area of your life. *Here is where the journey begins...*

Allow me to turn back the pages of time some 30-plus years ago when I was conceived in the womb to a mother who wanted to abort me and ended up using me, and to a father who left and neglected me. There were also two brothers who didn't want me around and a sister who came after me whom I ended up raising like my own.

That was the building block that created the foundation I later stood on - a foundation that was cemented together by the glue I would call **rejection** and **fear**...a foundation I would have to choose to either have it destroy me or me destroy it.

Those were the thoughts and emotions that echoed through my mind the first 18 years of my life. They left me emotionally scarred, almost to the point of being crippled.

Lifting the Weight: The Journey to Total Freedom

Every good relationship I had was affected by my inability to love, trust, and even forgive. It wasn't the other person, though; it was me. I allowed my emotions to control me to the point that they always placed me on a cycle I could not seem to break. The end result was the same, whether it was a high school friend or a family member. **The only constant contributing factor was me!**

Later in my life, I married and gave birth to two beautiful children who helped show me the meaning of unconditional love. I was also shown what I did not have as a child…and an adult. After having my second child, tipping the scale at 320 pounds, and encountering a health attack against my family, I knew it was time to make a change.

The doctors told me my husband had Cancer, my 12-week-old daughter picked up Aphomia, and my two-year-old son was autistic. My life was falling apart at the seams. Then came a divine intervention that saved my life by letting me know I had to change it. I started running and changed my diet. After a while, I lost the weight: 100 pounds **GONE**! I felt like a whole, new woman - but I was still broken. For one of the first times in my life, I was physically well, but emotionally disabled.

It is my firm belief that the weight I carried physically was a result of the weight I carried emotionally. It manifested its way through in an unhealthy way. The mass on my body was merely a reflection of my mental state.

320 pounds was simply a cry for help...a silent cry that nobody heard and one I did not openly express.

See, I was not eating because I wanted to be full. I was eating because I was "empty". The false sense of a full stomach gave me a sense of satisfaction that was short-lived.

How would I end the cycle?

How would the weight be lifted?

How could I change the outcome of my life that was ravaged by fear and rejection that left a slew of relationships wounded in the dust?

Here comes one of the **HARDEST** things I have ever done...

Lifting the Weight: The Journey to Total Freedom

Step One: I had to confront and acknowledge my fears. I had to determine what I contributed to them as well. I could no longer pretend I could not find my way and didn't know my way out of that dark, lonely hole I was in. Just like an alcoholic, I was addicted to the pain. I needed to change. It was then I realized: In order to change the fruit of a thing, I had to change the root of that thing. The fruits I was bearing were hurt, pain, and shame. I wanted joy, love, and peace! Confronting my past left me emotionally-intoxicated. I was disoriented, but speaking with a sober tongue. I hurt. I cried. I asked "*Why?*" to the ghosts of my past. I did not deserve it and decided right then that I would not keep it.

Holding on to it was killing me. Letting it go would set me free!

Step Two: I had to forgive. I had to turn back the clock over 30 years and forgive each and every single person who hurt me, scarred me, rejected me, abandoned me, and did not love me. No, I did not call each and every one of them; I spoke from my heart what I would have told them to their face - given the opportunity. I realize "hurt people...hurt people", but the cycle ends here. I will no longer contribute to hurting people. I am dedicated to helping them heal mentally, physically, and emotionally.

Step Three: I had to put reinforcements in place and retrain my emotions to respond different ways when placed in a situation that had an undertone of rejection or could create fear. I could not reach for the fork and plate. I could no longer allow myself to sabotage anymore relationships. I had to find a way. At three years old, it was okay for me to throw temper-tantrums - kicking, screaming, and crying until I got my way. At the age of 32, that is unacceptable. I had to remind myself daily of who **GOD** says I am in His Word. I confess His Word over my life daily. See, it's not enough to read His Word; you must *SPEAK IT.* His Words are life, and they will come to pass.

Lifting the Weight: The Journey to Total Freedom

What I want you to know is that beauty - true beauty - is not a look or feeling. It is the knowledge of who you are. The only way to come into that knowledge is to see yourself in His Word as He says it, believing His Word to be true and everything/everyone else to be a lie. Day by day, I began to breathe. Day by day, I began to heal. Day by day I began to forgive. Day by day, I began to love. Some days are still a struggle. Some days, I still fall - but the battle is not determined in your falls; it's in your get-back-ups!

To the woman reading this piece of my story today: You don't have to stay in the place you're in. Yes, they hurt you, lied on you, talked about you, abandoned you, molested you, scarred you, beat you, and violated you...but only **YOU** can free *YOU*. Take the exchange that was paid for **YOU** over 2,000 years ago by Christ shedding His blood on the cross at Calvary. Use that pain as power. Don't allow the enemy to make you feel mentally crazy when you are spiritually sane. Realize that you tried to fight it your way and lost; but I assure you, if you try it **GOD'S** way, you will *WIN*!

Now that we have dealt with the root of that thing, you can change the fruit of that thing!

Presented By Sherell Brown

I'm praying God bring you healing, health, and hope into your world...**HIS** way.

Blessings!

Awaken Your Wellness
Shonda S. Caines

My past story is a part of me, but not all of who I am. By owning my story, I became whole, healthy, and happy. Therefore, I lifted the weight off of my shoulders and *awakened my wellness*.

At some point in my life, I got fed up...really fed up.

I know a lot of people say that over and over, but this time was different.

As a freshman, I quickly realized almost everyone on my campus had family that lived within a few hours away, while my family was hours away on a plane ride. Being in a new city alone with that knowledge can be scary for a young 18-year-old.

I was comforted by the following:

1. My dad's mantra: *"Shonda, you know your dreams; make decisions that align with them."*

2. My goal was to **NOT** become a college statistic and **NOT** to succumb to the statistics associated with Black women.

3. Returning home was not an option. Being an older child and the first girl came with plenty of responsibilities. As a child reared in the Caribbean, the responsibilities were tumultuous. For example, when my American roommate's parents were still taking care of her laundry, for me - after around 12 years old - I had major responsibilities. In the Caribbean, our parents expected us to have started or finished dinner by the time they returned home after their long day. Naturally, it was expected that the responsibilities increased with age.

I quickly realized academics were my way to freedom. I grew up overweight as a child and physically developed sooner than I would have wanted to. Those factors led to inappropriate gestures and unwelcomed attention by neighborhood males. I was ready to lift the weight in so many ways before the age of 18. I took my secondary studies seriously. It was my top priority to "get away".

Lifting the Weight: The Journey to Total Freedom

During my pre-college medical examination, I weighed 207 pounds at the age of 18. **OUCH!** After spending many years going to the gym trying to lose weight with a neighbor of mine, I was well aware of my weight 'situation'. All of the other students seemed so slim.

Somehow, 19 years later, it's still a very vivid memory of mine...

Once I got a handle on college life, eating healthier options and exercising were on my radar. These two things were already ingrained in me from the cabbage soup diets and numerous nights at the gym as a teenager. Healthier food options were chosen and several days met **ME** at the gym.

Unfortunately, that wasn't enough. My choices weren't aligned with losing weight. A few years after receiving my undergraduate degree, I revisited the idea of graduate school - and losing weight. Neither were pursued. It was not until my sister visited two years after graduation when everything changed. We both found out that childhood abuse had occurred to us - in the same house. However, neither of us know about the other's abuse. Though she's younger than I am, she inadvertently empowered me to "lift the weight". All of those terrible episodes of sleepwalking and talking in my sleep had a source. She helped me put everything together through her bravery and the sharing of her story.

It broke my heart that during my own abuse nightmare, I was unable to protect her. *As the older sibling, I was supposed to protect her, right?* I fell short, and it pierced my heart terribly. During that Summer, letters were written, truths were exposed, and a weight was lifted.

Fast-forward to Winter of 2004...

Lifting the Weight: The Journey to Total Freedom

I was reinspired to apply for graduate school and pick back up my house-hunting journey. The weight of the childhood trauma was lifted and led to the confidence and empowerment needed to believe it was possible to not only pursue a graduate degree with a stressful full-time career, but also successfully complete an accelerated track - **AND** lose the excess physical weight...

Which is why I was fed up.

I was fed up with nurses assuming my medical stats would be higher than they were based on my body composition and weight. Thankfully, the plague of heart disease wasn't a hereditary threat.

I needed to eat healthier and consistently be active. **PERIOD.** At the age of 25, I decided it would be a devastation to allow ailments to become a part of my life and possibly affect my future legacy. I longed to take part in adult recreational sports. There were so many things (like physical activities) I had missed out on that I longed to experience. A contract was created and, when the ink dried, the work began.

Exercise? Diet? Mindset? Portion Control? Routine? Stress/Stressors?

While in graduate school, I was miraculously able to still thrive within my profession. Most days of the week, my schedule started at 8:00 a.m. and ended at 10:00 p.m. To achieve something never accomplished before, it was time to apply a new approach.

This time, it was different.

I had a friend of mine take my girth measurements and pictures to capture my wellness journey. Homeownership was accomplished - just as I had planned. With the responsibilities that came with homeownership - on top of the demands of an accelerated graduate program and stressful job - it was imperative that I be creative. With this information staring me in my face and the self-to-self contract in hand, a "how" had to be crafted. I knew it was not realistic nor healthy to believe any sane person was going to fit in a healthy diet and workout plan on top of this crazy self.

Well, at least in my mind and having failed at staying the course numerous times before, it had to be feasible.

Lifting the Weight: The Journey to Total Freedom

So, knowing that a successful and long-term weight-loss program required healthier food choices and exercise, I had to pick one while in graduate school. I chose food. My emphasis was not only on healthy food choices as a vegetarian, but doing research to find healthier versions of what I was eating, learning about portion sizes, reading food labels, exploring herbs and spices, the importance of water consumption, and feeding my body on a cellular level.

By nature, I am intrigued by new information. I love to do research, enjoyed peer review journals, and found myself drawn to a more natural *(and common sense)* approach of doing things. So, once that decision was made, it released a burden off of my shoulders. Prior to this acceptance and final decision, I was stagnant in this area of my life.

I was jumping into unchartered waters. No one in any network of mine had ever successfully lost weight and/or kept it off. A big "AH-HA" moment was finding out that on average, one slice of bread is a serving. Yikes! *How many of you knew that little secret?* For me, that bread revelation opened my eyes in so many ways. After beginning to research food, portion control, and food label reading, my eyes were stuck open!

For someone who wasn't exercising, I was well above my daily caloric intake. That led to increased weight and the inability to lose weight. In order to lose weight, we must consume less calories than we burn (in laymen's terms). Exercise - both cardio and weight-bearing - along with a sensible meal plan, are a must for success.

A goldmine within reach was discovered while I was at work. After taking on a new position a few years ago, and now in a space to exercise, I found a gym there. I absorbed every nutrition tidbit I could find, from magazines to nutrition journals.

I decided to make more health-conscious meals, increase my veggie intake, eat more protein, and be mindful of my portion sizes. Many aren't aware, but it's still possible to take in too many calories while eating healthier foods. I loaded my life with fresh whole foods and ate several snacks and meals per day. Once foods were discovered that worked for my body and journey, I kept them in rotation.

Lifting the Weight: The Journey to Total Freedom

I loved eating vegetable and Asian stir-fry. I ditched the sauce that came with the frozen veggies and added vegan protein. Upping my water consumption was huge, too. It's important to note: My last meal of the day was just before class began. This ensured I had adequate food to power through the accelerated classes after a long and demanding work day.

Once home, I oftentimes had a light snack before bed. School stretched me, but I finished with honors and had to face the second part of my self-to-self contract: incorporating exercise. I started the next day after my last class, but got fully serious after graduation in October after my family who flew in to celebrate with me had left.

So, it was just me, myself, and that darn contract. From there, I revisited the gym in the pit of the building. I started out with just cardio seven days a week, then added in free weights to my routine in the Fall of 2006. Once my birthday came around in February, I was fitting into jeans once too tight just six months prior.

During the colder months, the progress was very slow. As an Islander, I love the warmth of the sun on my body and long days. With the warmer temps, daylight savings, and my department in a new department, my weight loss shifted. We now had an upgraded gym, and I was minutes away from my previous apartment complex that had a state-of-the-art fitness facility.

So, you know what I did, right?

I used **every** opportunity possible to retreat to the empty onsite gym on my lunch break. With all the free time in the evenings with school completed, I spent it walking around the bustling developments happening in my old stomping grounds. Within a few months, I met employees from different departments who were also on their own weight-loss journeys. We looked forward to meeting up in the gym after work. I recall running for five minutes straight and returning the next day to ensure it wasn't a flux.

That was a beautiful moment.

Lifting the Weight: The Journey to Total Freedom

After months of staying focused and dedicated to my self-to-self contract, I was invited to join a weight-loss challenge, and did so. I had just a few more pounds to go, and figured it would get me there within 12 months of adding in my exercise.

I met the goal within 11 months!

My heaviest weight was 229 pounds.
I lost a total of 90 pounds and went from
a size 22 to a size 2 in 11 months!

This experience forced me to realize anything is possible. From here on out, I always, **ALWAYS** reference this very groundbreaking and intimate journey. It made me a stronger person in all areas of my life. I awakened a level of self-confidence that never existed before - so much so, I confidently negotiated various jobs at my house, asked for raises at work, took on new adventures (like running, weight-lifting, and swimming), and show up in a more authentic way.

I found out running came natural for me and tackled the fear of drowning by becoming a triathlete in 2012. Learning to swim and my weight-loss journey are, indeed, the two biggest self "projects" taken on that helped awaken the dormant Shonda. During my weight-loss 5th anniversary, I trained for my first half-marathon and traveled internationally solo to reflect and praise God.

I find a way to challenge my mental and physical capability and took it up a notch in 2015 by running my first 50-mile marathon. I've gone from daydreaming on the couch about losing weight, to signing up to run a 50-mile ultra-marathon to think about and see how the body reacts. I've been blessed since Fall of 2007 to travel around the world and test my physical and mental limitations. Now that I'm nearing my 10th weight-loss anniversary in Fall of 2017, I'm already pondering how I'd love to celebrate.

It's been a journey - to say the least. In the process, my passion was birthed. My pain was exposed. No longer dormant are my interests, talents, and gifts. I'm now the Founder of Awaken Your Wellness, LLC, Founder of EBN's Vegan Cuisine, LLC, and the Chief Fitness Officer of Shonda S. Caines.

Lifting the Weight: The Journey to Total Freedom

This journey allowed me to create and combine the areas necessary to awaken one's wellness. It does require an internal audit of what's weighing you down.

For those reading my story of *"Awakening My Wellness"*, I wanted to share with you some simple, yet practical steps needed to begin the process.

1. Determine if you have "weight" to release. If so, what are they and why?

2. Who is a part of the "weight" and what can be done to release him or her?

3. Is it realistic and what's a reasonable timetable?

4. What happens if the releasing process doesn't go as planned?

5. Who is your support team and how can they assist you during this time?

6. What area of the "weight" is most challenging and why?

7. Is there any area of the "weight" that can be tackled and released without external interactions? If it's a "weight" that deals with food, can you identify the root of the problem? Are you an emotional eater? Are there certain times, places, and things that cause you to emotionally eat? If so, can you pinpoint why? If not, are you open to seeking professional assistance to expose the cause(s)?

8. What, if any, lies have you been told and now believe as your truth? Make a list. Have any of them served you any good in the past 12 months? If not, why do you still believe them?

9. What is your relationship with food? Are you hung up on eating the same foods and food groups? Are you open to new food groups and healthier foods during this journey of lifting the weight and awakening your wellness?

It starts with who stares back at you in the mirror. Once we become fed up, our actions will follow...loudly. I encourage you to create a self-to-self contract like I did. I was so fed up with being unhappy in this area of my life, my contract didn't **NEED** to be written. It was said verbally and engrained in my soul.

Lifting the Weight: The Journey to Total Freedom

Hire someone to help you - if necessary. Seek out inspiration from suitable sources and find someone whose story is relatable. Empty your home of unhealthy foods if you can. Find healthier versions of what you eat. Understand that a gym membership isn't needed to begin. Determine who you can assign as your accountability partner - and pick at least to people. Make sure they're also progressing in life and are eager to assist. This partnership shouldn't be a burden on any level. If you follow my process and/or journey in any way and require assistance, please reach out to a professional in your area that will challenge you in any way. Now is the perfect time to Awaken Your Wellness and lift the weight that has for far too long weighed you down.

This is the most important thing: Lifting the Weight and Awakening Your Wellness is not a New Year's resolution, seasonal fad, or ego journey. It must be a decision birthed from a place you wish to detach from...a yearning that evokes a new beginning that is found within the depth of your beautiful soul. Join me on an endless journey of awakening our wellness as women.

You **ARE** worth it!

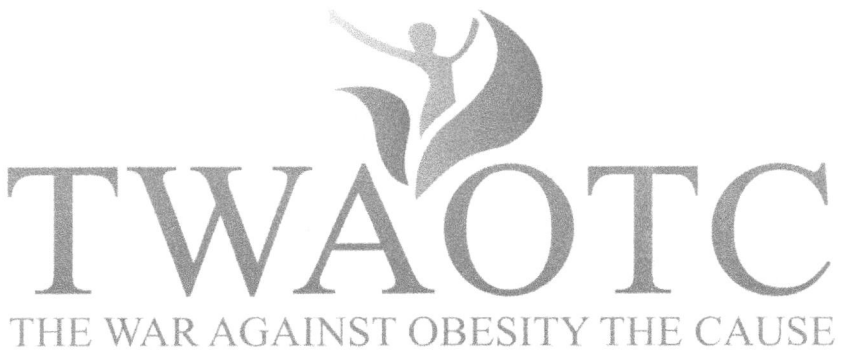

TWAOTC

THE WAR AGAINST OBESITY THE CAUSE

Dead Weight to Manifested Dreams
Zipporah Gamble

By now, you should've already read the title of this chapter. It has probably left you a bit perplexed, as you may not understand exactly what it means or where exactly I am going with those words. Well, I promise you this: Before the end of this chapter, you will fully understand what *Dead Weight to Manifested Dreams* entails.

Many of you may be just like me, in that you inherited dead weight upon your life the moment you were conceived. As a young girl, I was raised in a single parent home by a mother who always worked. It's not the life she had hoped for, but she did whatever she had to do to ensure we had a roof over our heads, food on the table, and clothes on our backs. My mother is a very strong woman who gave me all she had to give. However, our mother-daughter relationship was anything but normal.

Presented By Sherell Brown

I imagine in most homes, the mother would sit down with her daughter and talk to her about all of the challenges she would encounter in life - from puberty, to boys, to sex. Well, I never had **any** of those conversations with my mother. Due to her not receiving those talks in *her* youth, her concern was that she would tell me the wrong information. I learned the majority of what I know about the maturation process of a female by picking up on what my friends would say and do, in conjunction with the educational classes my mother would sign me up for at school.

I gave you that insight as to how I gained knowledge of becoming a woman so that you could capture me in the midst of these intricate moments of my life. I ask that you reach down within yourself and make the connection with your inner-child while we rest here for a moment to explore my conflicted mind…

Lifting the Weight: The Journey to Total Freedom

Now, as you make the connection, your mind may take you back to the life that was presented to *you* as a child. I know there are many of you who may have endured more hardships and pains than I have, and my heart goes out to you. I was a confused girl who really didn't know who she was. The image I had of myself was so obscure, the person I saw in the mirror did not reflect the image I had in my mind. Today, I can look at pictures of myself from back then with my husband who says, "*Girl, you were a dime-piece!*" I could not be convinced back then that I was beautiful. The reason I couldn't see my own beauty was due to something which may sound so innocent; nonetheless, it had such a damaging impact on my life.

I was bullied and picked on by boys. Those boys **terrorized** me to the point of me having internal trauma no one could even see. I was harassed so bad, I felt like I began to die inside. I can't even mention some of the names or things they used to say about me... The pain hurt so bad, but I never shared it with anyone. I had family and friends who were there in my life, but I didn't trust anyone to help me handle my brokenness. If my inside was displayed on the outside, I would be a massacred mess - completely unrecognizable.

I know some of my family and friends who may read this book never knew what I was going through and the searing effect it had on my life. Whatever those boys said about me, I believed them. Those words were some of the first words I'd even had spoken over me in reference to my appearance and worth - which brings me to my point:

We, as parents, have to ensure we are speaking words of affirmation over our children because the life we **DON'T** speak may be the death someone else speaks. The question you need to stop and ask yourself is this:

Am I speaking life over my children or spouse? Or am I leaving that for someone else to do?

Contrary to popular belief, words carry power. In most cases, we don't even comprehend how much power **ONE** word carries. A word has the power to change your entire life - if you believe it, be it good or bad.

Lifting the Weight: The Journey to Total Freedom

The words those boys spoke over me caused many internal wounds. One thing about internal wounds is they seem to take even longer to heal. Not being able to visually see the wound does not enable you to know exactly how to approach it. I did not know why those boys disliked me. I never gave them a reason to gain pleasure from causing my feelings pain. I was never told by anyone that boys may pick on you simply because they like you. Some of the boys who bullied me did so because they had insecurities of their own that rendered them incapable of simply stepping up to me to voice how they truly felt about me. Other boys had different reasons all their own, such as the conquest to be "the one" to take my virginity.

Needless to say, they were **ALL** unsuccessful in their attempts, which made them the most malicious ones of all. Their pride was hurt, so they would use their popularity, influence, and their weapon of choice (their tongue) to destroy me.

Presented By Sherell Brown

My being a Spartan Doll (a dance team member of our award-winning Campbell Middle School marching band) and a member of our award-winning chorus mattered to me during this time. All that mattered was how I would now view everyone's perception of me. I believed everyone saw me as this fat, chubby, ugly girl the boys spoke of. If you saw pictures of me from when those boys rallied together to attack me, you wouldn't understand how I could ever succumb to believe such heinous lies, especially when the very essence of my biblical name, Zipporah, means *"Beauty"*.

I believe I failed to mention I grew up as an only child whose father was basically nonexistent in my life. I lacked self-esteem and confidence since I didn't have my father present in my life to validate my beauty and help establish my self-worth. Two of the most dangerous things in this world are not knowing who you are and how much you're worth. I must emphasize how vitally important it is for young boys **and** girls to have a good male father-figure or role model in their lives to demonstrate day in and day out how a woman should be treated.

Lifting the Weight: The Journey to Total Freedom

Another point of view to consider is the negative behaviors that are modeled before them. As a result of my father's absence from my life, my mother was left to shoulder the load on her own. In the midst of all the strength it took to be the sole provider, we lost those soft and tender moments I so desperately needed from my mother. I never confided in her or ever took thought to solicit her advice pertaining to the issues and struggles I faced. I guess the reason I never considered my mother to pour my heart into was because it was never made known to me that she was an option.

During my senior year in high school, I met the man who is now my husband. At the time, I almost doubled my weight from my freshman year. After high school, my husband entered the military, joining the U.S. Army. This was another difficult time in my life, as we had spent nearly every day together...until that point. He would be apart from me until he completed all of his basic *and* advanced training. We could be together again once he was assigned to his permanent duty station.

During the six-month span when he was in training, we were able to see each other a couple of times. When it was all said and done, I weighed about 250+ pounds on my 5' 4" frame and size 6 1/2 feet. I had gained 50 to 60 pounds since my husband last saw me. This was a difficult thing for him to see me in such a state. The image engraved in my mind of myself all of those years ago had finally manifested itself to my outward being. I would soon begin recognizing a disconnect between us.

The way he used to look at me with desire...he didn't look at me that way anymore. There was a stiff and fridge coldness that rose up between us. I remember some of the hardest times being when we would go shopping for clothes. It would take me forever to find something in my size. I would put on something and ask my husband for his opinion. His face would speak before his mouth would utter a word. There was nothing spoken verbally nor nonverbally that would indicate he was intrigued in the least.

Lifting the Weight: The Journey to Total Freedom

I remember at some point him telling me he was no longer happy. I asked what his reason for his unhappiness was, and although we had many conversations (and arguments) about my weight, it was not the primary reason why he felt so angry and betrayed by me. He asked me, *"How can you be happy with somebody and truly love that person when they're not even happy nor in love with themselves?"*

I was in such a deep state of depression from my emotional abuse, I had difficulty understanding. He went on. *"How can I call myself a real man and be happy when I know you're in pain? My happiness comes from knowing you're happy and you feel as though you're the greatest woman on earth."*

My husband did his best to motivate me in the ways that he knew how. He began working out with me at the gym, among other things like running or walking the track. He brought me different workout equipment, too. However, none of his methods worked - partially due to his militant demeanor and because I had buried myself so deep in a pit of misery and anguish until I didn't know how to get out of it.

Isn't it crazy how we can go through a full day of work doing all kinds of different things, but internally, we have accomplished **nothing**? Just think: After we finish allowing ourselves to be entertained by our distractions, eventually we're going to find ourselves still stuck in our own realities.

For me, I would start to adhere to certain weight-loss regimens. I even got a membership at Curves. I lost a few pounds here and there, but nothing long-lasting. I remember being out with my husband one day and we ran into some of his fellow soldiers. They thought I was his *mother*. What a blow that was to my heart!

I did manage to lose about 30 pounds before we departed Fort Hood, Texas. I was ready for a new season in my life. I had been suffocating in that sorrow for too long. We had been married for six years and trying to conceive a child ever since we said "I do". In all of those years, it just never happened for us. It was time to seek some professional help to get to the bottom of the mystery.

Lifting the Weight: The Journey to Total Freedom

The specialist my doctor sent me to had uncovered an underlying benefactor towards my weight gain. **FINALLY,** after all of those years, I learned my body was working against me the entire time. I suffered from something called Polycystic Ovarian Syndrome (PCOS). PCOS is an issue that causes a woman's hormones to become imbalanced. It can produce problems with the menstrual cycle and make it almost impossible to get impregnated. PCOS may also cause unwanted changes in one's appearance, such as the growth of hair in unwanted places. If PCOS goes untreated for some time, eventually, it can cause serious health problems like diabetes and heart disease. Many small cysts begin to grow on the ovaries of most women with PCOS. Although there is presently no cure for PCOS, with the help of early detection and treatment, women can control the symptoms and prevent long-term issues.

All of that time - since puberty - I had been battling an enemy I did not know about, not to mention the demons I would later fight within my own mind. It has finally been revealed to me the dead weight that was trying to kill me softly.

Presented By Sherell Brown

From the moment I was conceived in my mother's womb, the odds were against me. Ever since I started having my periods, my discharge of blood would be very heavy, lasting for a full week. Besides the excess discharge, my cramps were *excruciating*. I didn't know any better. I thought all girls' menstrual cycles were consistent with mine. I was curious as to why my period didn't come on every month or for a couple of months at a time, but I never had enough courage to talk about my secrets with someone else.

Much of what I went through in life was preventable. You see, the dead weights I had to carry were once carried by my parents. My father came from a broken and dysfunctional home, which is why he was never able to be there for me. He didn't know how to be a good father. He never had his father there to set the example he needed to see. My mother didn't know the words to speak to me as a mother because she had not witnessed those things in her own life when she was a young girl. I can't be upset with my mother for not being able to give me something she never received herself. I recently found out my mother had PCOS as well, which is why she only gave birth to me - and she didn't even do that until she was 37 years old. My mother has also dealt with miscarriages, just as I have.

Lifting the Weight: The Journey to Total Freedom

Parents, let's be informative. We need to empower our children with the knowledge to be successful, having as little dead weight (baggage) to carry as possible on their journey through this life. It would've been a blessing for me to know then what I know now…

Well, we have an understanding of what dead weights are. Now, let us get to the manifested dreams.

Regardless of me knowing about the dead weights in my life, that alone could not get me to my manifested dreams. I still had to do what it took to get the weight off - and keep it off. I could not do anything until I received the mental and emotional healing I needed to mend my infected wounds.

Presented By Sherell Brown

In times past, I tried to shed my weight for the wrong person and for all the wrong reasons. I tried to lose the weight for my husband, which was the wrong answer. I entered our marriage wounded and broken. I depended on my husband to mend my wounds. Though my husband is a wise, anointed, and appointed man of God, my 'situation' was something I had to give to my Father in Heaven. I had to take all of my tears and wash His feet with them. I made the mistake of depending on my husband more than God. God taught me a lesson through the attacks and battles launched at our union - things that almost shipwrecked our marriage.

It's time for us (as believers) to be real and authentic. We have to take off the mask and makeup, and come before the throne of grace broken and humble - regardless of who may be in the midst. We need to lay down our titles and pride, and prove to God we are not afraid nor ashamed to show Him our true, messed up, and broken selves. We've been presented this false truth that we, as believers, don't go through depression or have mental breakdowns...but we do. Once I gave God my all, I received my total healing.

Lifting the Weight: The Journey to Total Freedom

You see, because the damage was done internally, I had to receive my healing internally before anyone could see the new transformation of my inside on the outside. I was able to achieve the outward transformation by doing something different. We can't do the same thing and expect to get different results. I was introduced to a company by the name of Herbalife. This entailed me replacing two of my meals with a protein shake and a healthy meal for dinner. Now, that is **NOT** a route you have to take. It was my jumpstart for me.

Since lifting the weight, I have lost 55 pounds to date. I have been blessed with **two** beautiful baby boys, Houston and Jordan, who are two of my manifested dreams.

My life has been forever changed.

"LIFTING THE WEIGHT" CONCLUSION

"Our life is a sum total of the choices we have made". If nothing else, take away from reading this book that no matter what circumstance or situation life throws at you, you have a **choice**. You have a **choice** to accept it or reject it. You have the **choice** to change it or conform to it. **You have a choice.**

The authors of this book shared with you firsthand what life has dealt them - from poor self-image to molestation - and how it manifested physically in their health and with their bodies. We can never promise you the hard lessons won't come, but the truth is the only way out is *through*. We have to walk **through** our processes, take each lesson learned, be healed from it, learn to love in it, and grow through it. Otherwise, we will never be *fully* free.

Your freedom and the life you desire starts with you exposing the root cause that has held you bound, expelling it from your life and being empowered with the knowledge that you are **more** than an overcomer. Remember: **Every** journey starts with a single step. Today can be the day yours begins.

Lifting the Weight: The Journey to Total Freedom

Meet the Authors

Compiler and Weight-Lifter / Sherell Brown

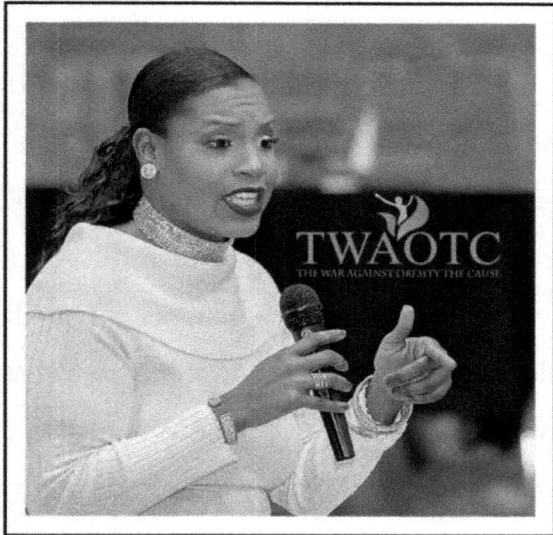

Presented By Sherell Brown

Sherell Brown is a 'Category Creator' in the Health and Wellness arena, combining a mix of both professional skills and personal experiences that produces results. She has worked with persons from all walks of life, helping them to achieve their personal goals and, ultimately, creating a better quality of life.

Sherell is the C.E.O. of Sherell Brown Health Concierge Services, the Publisher of *"L.O.S.E." Health & Wellness Magazine*, Best-Selling Author of *The Blueprint to Weight Loss: The Truth Revealed,* and a sought-after Radio Personality. She has spearheaded campaigns such as "The Bra Out", a fundraiser designed to bring awareness to Breast Cancer in the Island of Abaco, Bahamas, where she also held aerobic sessions and went on to launch other campaigns, to include "Team No Rolls" and "Lose with Me". As the Founder of 'The War Against Obesity The Cause', she is teaching people how to eat to live and not to die!

Lifting the Weight: The Journey to Total Freedom

Sherell has consulted and motivated thousands of people across the globe by transforming their lives. When speaking with her, she will tell you her favorite part of the transformation process is the smile that appears *"when the diamond within an individual is unearthed, and what they knew was always on the inside is now glistening on the outside"*.

Most importantly, Sherell provides education and tools to help ensure the success of your journey. She has dedicated her life to helping others become healthier while teaching them how to reprogram their minds towards food and how to reset one's metabolism. No matter where you are in your health and wellness journey, Sherell is there to help you with her personal coaching and consulting.

Presently, Sherell resides in Murfreesboro, Tennessee with her husband, Desmond Brown, and her two children, young Master Seth and Princess Grace Brown.

With her love for the Lord and her relentless passion, Sherell is ready to serve you!

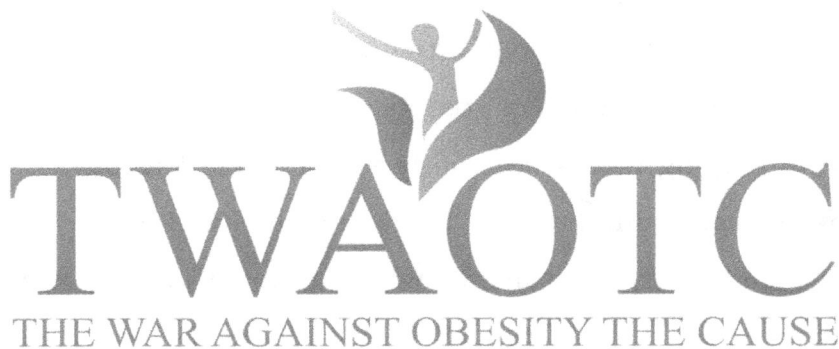

TWAOTC

THE WAR AGAINST OBESITY THE CAUSE

Lifting the Weight: The Journey to Total Freedom

Co-Author / Weight-Lifter Eboni Gee

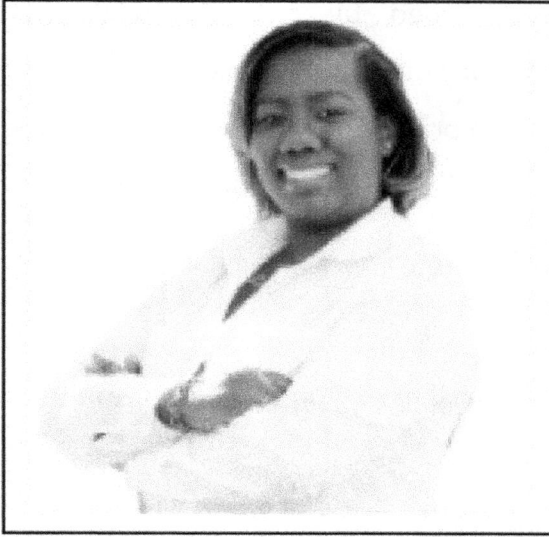

Presented By Sherell Brown

Eboni Gee is a wife, mother, and Registered Nurse. Her passion is helping people who are looking to make peace with their past mistakes, regrets, and bad decisions so that they can turn those lessons into blessings and live in their purpose. This is accomplished by creating healthy self-care and personal development routines to facilitate one's transformation to bring about a peace and harmony to life that is irreplaceable. Eboni's purpose is to help nurture the passions of others so that they can find the purpose that is waiting for them.

To Travis and Tariq: Thank you for your support.

Lifting the Weight: The Journey to Total Freedom

Co-Author / Weight-Lifter Iris Hernandez

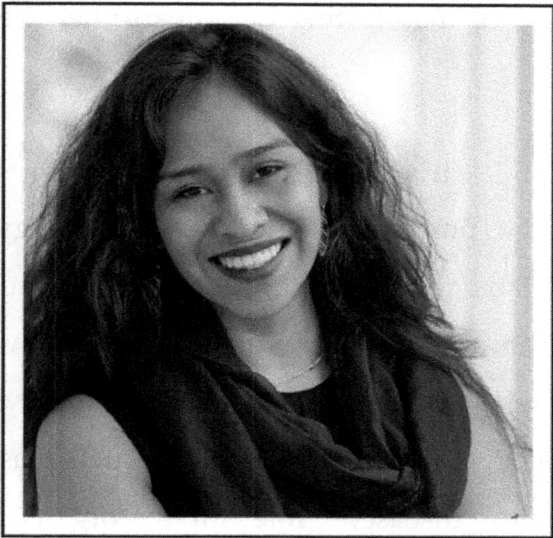

Presented By Sherell Brown

Iris Hernandez was born in Mexico City and moved to the United States at the age of 10. She grew up using herbs and home remedies, as her family encouraged the use of natural medicine. Her initial goal was to become a medical doctor, but in the process of manifesting her dream, her life took a big turn.

At the age of 19, Iris began to study Quantum Physics and discovered the power of God's healing energy. She later realized the damage of pharmaceuticals and chose to continue her career through natural healing. She is now a Holistic Practitioner who helps her community in many ways. She has helped clients with imbalances such as diabetes, cardiovascular disease, infertility, organ or gland malfunctions, depression, hyperactivity, physical disconnect, emotional damage, and more.

Iris is a firm believer of Christ and the healing power of the Holy Spirit. She gives all credit to GOD and continues her walk by encouraging others to worship GOD through the proper maintenance of their physical body, soul, and spirit (1 Thessalonians 5:23). She knows that in order to allow GOD to live within, we must keep the temple clean.

Lifting the Weight: The Journey to Total Freedom

"Don't Die of a Broken Heart" (Isaiah 61:1) was developed by GOD through Iris as a campaign to encourage and teach others about the correlation of mind, body, emotions, and spiritual health and how each affects the heart.

With GOD's guidance, Iris would like to continue to teach not only about health (3 John 2), but also spread JESUS CHRIST's unlimited love through HIS WORD via "GOD is Love Ministries" (Mark 12:30-31).

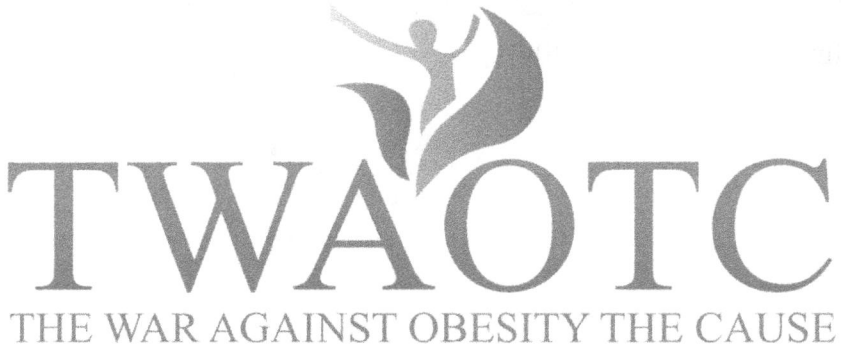

TWAOTC

THE WAR AGAINST OBESITY THE CAUSE

Lifting the Weight: The Journey to Total Freedom

Co-Author / Weight-Lifter Shonda S. Caines

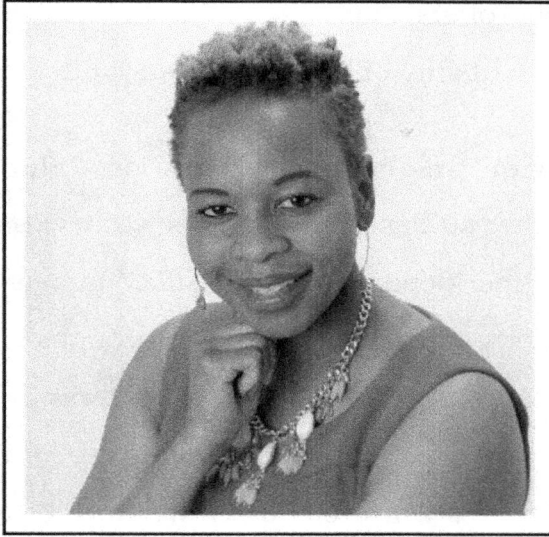

Presented By Sherell Brown

Shonda S. Caines is a Wellness Catalyst, Fitness Chef, Speaker, and Author. After her own journey to awakening her health and wellness, she strives to empower women to maximize their health and fitness potential. Through specialized programs, she offers tools, tips, and strategic plans to help clients obtain a quality of life via a holistic approach.

Speaking with an entrancing passion, Shonda ignites (transforms) her audience with concise strategies and models that extend the depths of their subconscious to expose, address, reverse, and harvest breakthroughs. Besides her professional and real-life personal experiences, her infectious personality, undeniable passion, and "keep it real" humor births a boundless sense of power within the lives she has been called to serve. The outcome is a generational breakthrough that takes clients and their families from merely 'existing' to 'thriving' via an Awakened Transformation.

Lifting the Weight: The Journey to Total Freedom

Equipped with her MPA, Fitness Nutrition Specialization, Weight Loss Specialization, Certified Personal Training credentials from the National Academy of Sports Science, Group Exercise Instructor Certification, RRCA Run Coach Certification, nine-year 90-pound weight loss lifestyle, seven years helping individuals maximize their quality of life, and 21 years of personal real-life experiences, Shonda is qualified to be empathic, meet her clients and audiences where they are, and help them expose the transparency needed to develop trust and provide structured programs - ones that yield results.

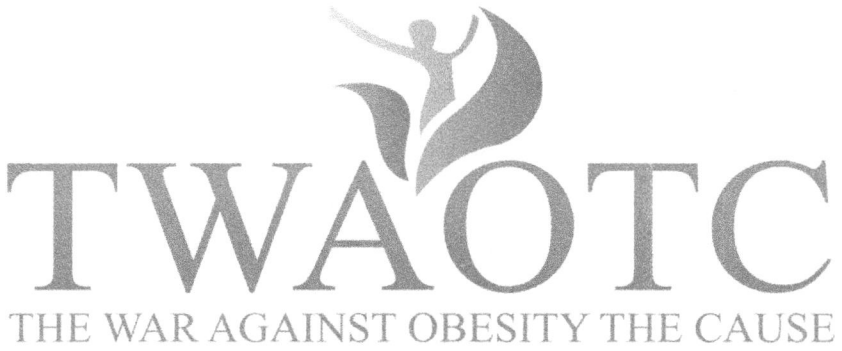

TWAOTC

THE WAR AGAINST OBESITY THE CAUSE

Lifting the Weight: The Journey to Total Freedom

Co-Author / Weight-Lifter Zipporah Gamble

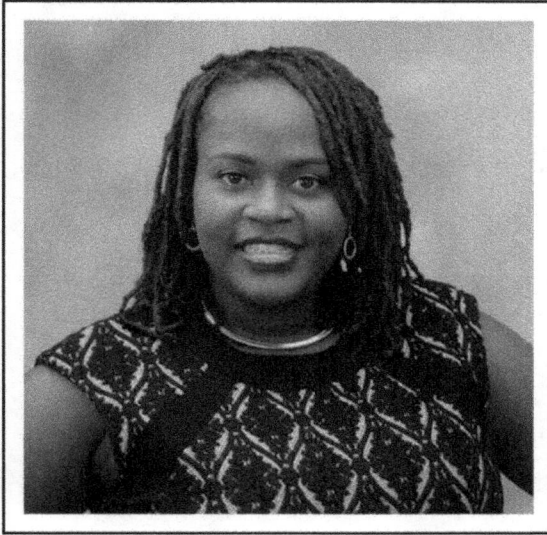

Presented By Sherell Brown

Zipporah Juaneek Gamble had the pleasure of growing up in the beautiful state of Florida. Her passion for healthcare shines as bright as the sun itself.

Zipporah is a Certified Phlebotomist and received her Bachelor of Science in Nursing from the University of Saint Mary, Kansas. Also, being a military spouse affords her the opportunity to understand how mental, emotional, and physical traumas can place individuals in a captivity that is not their own.

There's nothing Zipporah enjoys more than helping and healing others. The only thing that precedes her love for her family and her passion for healthcare is her relationship with God.

www.ingramcontent.com/pod-product-compliance
Lightning Source LLC
Chambersburg PA
CBHW071241020426
42333CB00015B/1575